Twilight Request

By Margo P. Cohen, M.D.

Contents

TWILIGHT REQUEST	1
THE FIRSTAFTER	2
THE BIGGER PICTURE	4
SINS OF OMISSION	6
GETTING TO SURGERY	11
FALSE OPTIMISM	14
THE ONCOLOGIST PRONOUNCES	15
OTHER OPTIONS	19
A SEARCH FOR MEANING	20
SIDE EFFECTS	22
INTERCURRENT PROBLEMS - DR. SOUP APPEARS	24
RELAPSE	26
DR. SLOBBER ARROGANTLY PREVAILS	28
WHEN IT RAINS IT POURS	30
RESPITE	31
SETBACK	32
PREVARICATIONS AND OBFUSCATIONS	34
WAITING	36
HIDDEN EVIL	38
CHANGE OF COURSE	39
BADGERING	41
ACQUIESCENCE	45
FAILURE	48
MORE INATTENTIVENESS	51

THE WIFE	53
THE HUSBAND	56
MENS SANA	58
AND SO IT GOES	60
NOT A DREAM	62
RADIATION	63
TO REHAB AND BACK	65
OTHER UNDERLINGS	67
THE REIGNING QUEEN	69
NO RECOURSE	73
WHAT OTHERS SAY	77
DONE WITH HIM	78
REFLECTIONS	79
AFTER	81
FROM ON HIGH	83
Definitions	86

Chapter 1

TWILIGHT REQUEST

Actuarial statistics say the life expectancy for a man of 73 is another 24 years. In early December on his 73rd birthday my husband Perry had a radical prostatectomy for what turned out to be an aggressive prostate cancer. The interval between diagnosis and death was a scant two years. Not fair, not fair at all. Such a bad disease in such a good man, who asked me, before his morphine-induced twilight, to chronicle how he went from health to his final breath, under the travesty of medical care at a famous cancer hospital.

Chapter 2

THE FIRSTAFTER

Perry played vigorous tennis the day before surgery. He showed no sign of fear, yet he was enormously happy to discover that I, not an angel, was caressing him in the recovery room. Walking into his hospital room that evening I found him on his cell phone placing calls in rapid succession, conversing animatedly with whoever was on the other end, exclaiming that he felt terrific. Propped up in bed with an IV running, a tube from the wound unremittingly filling the drainage bag, his lower abdomen swathed in dressings, and his legs enveloped in pressurized wrappings, he seemed not only oblivious to any discomfort but also a bit euphoric.

How remarkably well he's doing! I thought, until he mentioned that he had taken an IV push of his pain med shortly before my arrival. I realized that he was on a fentanyl high.

Perry reverted to a less conversational mode in the days following his discharge, suffering from elephantiasis of the scrotum. The hospitalization was the minimal two days, the key to discharge being ambulation, eating, and slowing of flow into the drain so that it could be pulled – but they didn't tell him that the fluid in the operative field had to go someplace when the drain was pulled - and the path of least resistance was into the scrotum. Thus, the postoperative high was followed by a period of little patience with relatives and friends calling to ask how he was doing. He gave the minimal response, anxious to just get them off the phone. There are no words that make you feel better when you feel awful. He was happy to have come through the surgery and thought that he had been cured, he just wanted to get through this misery.

During the interval of restless nights after surgery, discomfited by the catheter in the first couple of weeks and by unexplained awakenings with a mysterious energy in the middle of the night, he took to his computer - digesting analyst reports, identifying stocks, reading and writing innumerable e-mails. He made stabs at lists of assets and access information for bank accounts, trading accounts, life insurance, and retirement accounts, apparently for me. These nocturnal activities may have reflected a renewed vigor in doing all the things that held interest for him. He continued to follow the markets and the news in areas of personal and mutual interest - the Middle East, health care, and the political and foreign affairs faux pas of the president - who he did not admire.

In the ensuing couple of months, the quiet reserved man I married, who a nephew once dubbed as "Uncle Taciturn," became increasingly talkative. I would overhear him describing to friends the details of his diagnosis, the operation, Gleason score, and risk category, and professing how well he was doing. The evening before his eight-week follow-up with the urologic surgeon he was telling friends and relatives what he and his surgeon believed - that the surgery was successful, the PSA was expected to be close to zero, and that periodic checking of the PSA would be all that was required. At the end of the follow-up exam the surgeon optimistically scheduled the next appointment four months down the road. But upon receiving the results that the PSA level was 11, he advised Perry to see a medical oncologist post haste.

Perry shared this bad news with whoever called, but his loquaciousness abruptly declined when the test results ordered by the oncologist were even less rosy. The bone scan showed foci of metastatic activity and the MRI showed iliac nodes and recurrence in the operative field. My husband's conversations became more guarded, merely reciting these findings.

Chapter 3

THE BIGGER PICTURE

I had ominous forebodings from the moment I read the report of the biopsy performed by his urologist, who he been seeing regularly for years. In medical terminology it described adenocarcinoma in both sides of the prostate, overall Gleason score of 8-9, and wicked cytological characteristics on immunostaining for prostate cancer markers, although no seminal vesicle involvement.

The MRI showed a tumor mass in the left lobe, suggesting that perhaps the biopsy sample from the right lobe reflected contamination of the needle with left lobe prostate tissue, and the bone scan was negative for metastatic lesions - giving soon to be dashed comfort.

Perry took the biopsy news in stride, not quite digesting its import, but knowing enough to be relieved at the findings of the MRI and bone scan. He waited with outward calm the call from the radiation therapist recommended by the urologist, who advised that this was the best treatment. He liked the sincere yarmulke-wearing man he met the second week in November, and was ready to embark on a course of radiation, preceded by a course of anti-androgen treatment which that same urologist *-whose clinical competence I came to doubt-* preparatory to radiation. Reading the results from the small Phase II study which the radiation therapist co-authored, and the larger Phase III multicenter study, I had second thoughts. Both studies showed that pretreatment with Lupron (the LHRH agonist that diminishes androgen production) improved outcome but the statistics for disease free interval and disease-specific deaths were far less favorable in men with Gleason scores of 8 or above, giving me nightly visions of spreading cancer cells as time passed until Lupron and then radiation took hold.

So we made an appointment for later that week with the head of urologic surgery at another hospital. This man rambled unhelpfully for close to an hour. Among other things, he said that he had just refused to operate on another man with similar findings, and that the man had begged and cried, and was the reason we had spent two hours in the waiting room. Then he asked Perry what his urologist had felt on rectal exam. "That's the funny thing," Perry replied, "I wondered why he didn't examine me and thought maybe he didn't like me". "What?" I blurted out, shocked. "He didn't do a rectal?" "He used to" said Perry, "but he stopped four or five years ago." I was speechless.

The surgeon took Perry into the next room for exam, returning a few moments later with a look of satisfaction. "That was enlightening" he said. "There's a big mass, but it's confined to one lobe. Maybe it's in the seminal vesicles but we can take those out. I can get around this in surgery." He then added, somewhat gleefully: "I don't think those lymph nodes are positive, they're mostly less than one centimeter which is almost always negative, a couple are more than one but less than two centimeters, which is almost always positive. Let's do a Prostascint scan to see if they light up and if they don't we can do surgery." He flashed a winning smile and said, "I'm pretty sure the scan will be negative, we can schedule you for surgery." And so he did.

Chapter 4

SINS OF OMISSION

How could a urologist, whose bread and butter trade is in rectal exams, fail to do one? I didn't doubt my husband's statement - a man would surely know whether a rectal exam had been performed. Documentation of this shocking omission by asking for the office record was a little tricky since we didn't want to alert the urologist of any specter of potential malpractice. When Perry called to request a copy of his record, saying that it would be helpful for consultations, the urologist first responded that there was no reason to do so, radiation therapy was the best option. When pressed, the urologist offered - if you want, you can come here and copy it, we don't have time for that. Once received, the record documented that the urologist had not performed a single rectal exam for the past 5 years. It also showed that the urologist had felt a hard nodule that had doubled in size in the year between the last rectal exams he had performed.

Oddly, the urologist was diligent in offering samples of Viagra and then Cialis and had written a note that he thought the latter was better than the former. I had never seen Perry taking either, but had observed him shuddering over TV ads warning to see one's doctor for erections lasting more than four hours. When I asked him about this, he said the urologist kept questioning if he liked Cialis, and so he said he did, to make him happy and stop him asking.

About a year after my husband's death I met the infamous urologist at a wedding in Colorado. I had engaged with him in casual conversation during the pre-wedding cocktail event about the merits of taking Diamox - which I had done - to forestall mountain sickness. He was dogmatically opinionated, a bit weird in his giant cowboy hat, and his face seemed familiar. I realized why the next day. Unable to resist when he commented that we had conversed the night before, I said that in fact we had been introduced previously. I told him my husband's name, adding: "He could not be here - you know why". The not-so-hidden message in this comment to the urologist was asking if it occurred to him that if he had performed regular rectal exams, would my husband's prostate cancer been detected at a curable stage.

In a New York Times column ruminating about the lost art of physical diagnosis, Abraham Varghese described a woman with shortness of breath and seizures, in whom scans, performed to rule out pneumonia, blood clots or stroke, showed metastatic lesions in the lungs and brain. These findings belatedly prompted a physical exam which revealed a breast mass that was visible to the naked eye, certainly palpable and for which no one had ever examined.

If the physician caring for my husband's brother Ronald, dead at age 49 of metastatic colon cancer and father of a ten-year-old son, had paid proper attention, would Ronnie have lived a longer life?

On the recommendation of his internist, Ronald had sought a gastroenterologist for abdominal discomfort after noticing rectal bleeding. The gastroenterologist delivered the innocuous diagnosis of hemorrhoids. I was retrospectively astounded that one of the most fundamental principles of the practice of medicine had been ignored. Simply by taking a history, the internist would have learned that Ronald's father died with metastatic carcinoma of the colon. Possibly, Ronald had even volunteered the information. Had appropriate attention been given to the family history, had the telling symptom been properly evaluated, the primary cancer might have been resected before seeding metastatically in the liver. At one point after identification of the primary lesion Ronald sarcastically asked me if I thought he should call the internist and let him know how the hemorrhoids had turned out. Ronald was referred to a local oncologist who offered standard chemotherapy with an old drug, oblivious that more aggressive approaches had evolved with regimens that entailed newer drugs and routes of administration and with which long term survivors had been reported. But how could Ronald know? How could anyone know without other counsel?

The patient, believing the authoritative voice, is buoyed with hope on hearing the proposed schedule of treatment - "A few hours a day, a few days a week, every few weeks for several months, we'll follow up every couple of months, etc. etc." - all cementing hope that he or she will be alive for follow-up.

Ronnie died at home in a hospital bed within a year, sedated and without pain or much cognizance. Perry witnessed his brother's end, confiding to me later how deeply etched that memory was, not knowing that he would die bedridden, albeit mercifully slipping into unconsciousness in his final days, with me and our sons present at his final breath.

If the gynecologist regularly visited by my sister Judy, dead at age 53, had performed a proper pelvic exam, would she have lived a longer life?

When she began noting urinary urgency and abdominal swelling, Judy promptly visited her gynecologist, who told her not to worry. He said her problem would be cured once he removed her uterine fibroids, which in fact were long-standing, benign, asymptomatic, and inconsequential. I listened to the gynecologist tell me of his astonishment at the totally unexpected operative findings, which showed a huge malignancy and metastatic foci in the abdomen. This from the man who completely ignored my sister's recent history and, unfathomably in a physician whose singular expertise was pelvic exams, missed the mass in the cul-de-sac that was undoubtedly palpable to even lesser experienced hands. The pathology report at the same well-known local hospital misread the nature of the cancer, and the wrong therapy was initiated. Judy died just one year after diagnosis - a year in which she endured a multitude of therapeutic strategies and interventions: ablative surgery, radiation, chemotherapy, thoracentesis to drain the malignant pleural effusions that compressed her lungs, paracentesis to alleviate the painful distension from weeping malignant lesions studding in her abdomen. Visiting her at home in her last days I avoided answering her question - could this end been averted by appropriate intervention? As Perry's disease progressed, remembering Ronnie and Judy, he must have asked himself the same question.

Missed physical findings in another family member had a blessedly favorable outcome. Some eight years after successful removal of a benign brain tumor my mother-in-law noticed stiffness and weakness in her arm and hand. She described it to me during a distressed phone call after an appointment with a neurologist. Confirming the opinion of an internist, he had informed her that her symptoms represented residual from the previous brain surgery, coupled with a large psychological overlay. She was so panicked and hysterical, felt so abandoned, that I, no angel - this was after all my mother-in-law - invited her to spend the night with us. I listened to her complaints and examined the bothersome hand. I immediately noted that the small muscles were atrophied and the reflexes were hyperactive, consistent with a spinal cord lesion.

The internist and neurologist had failed to do this simplest part of a physical exam directly related to the chief complaint.

I referred her to a neurosurgeon who performed a myelogram (this before MRIs and CAT scans were de rigueur) and post-haste scheduled surgery. He found an octopus of tumor surrounding the cervical cord with tentacles extending to the base of the brain. The neurosurgeon paged me from the operating room to let me know that the situation was inoperable. He wanted to ask me what I wanted to do in this sixty-eight-year-old woman, seeking my concurrence for simply closing the incision and not attempting resection. It was my unintended non-appearance at the time of her surgery that was my biggest contribution to this case. He told me the next day that when I hadn't responded to the page after an acceptable interval, he returned to the operative field, picking and dissecting and removing as much tumor as he could. He was a very good neurosurgeon. My mother-in-law was eighty-three when she died of unrelated disease.

Chapter 5

GETTING TO SURGERY

The Prostascint scan was calendared for the end of November, to be followed by a return visit to the surgeon the next day for his pronouncement on whether he would operate. The decision would be no if the scan showed any nodes lighting up since positive nodes affected outcome statistics and he had made it clear he would not want to chance a negative impact on his success record. The two-week wait for the scan was dismaying, two weeks of doing nothing, while my visions of spreading cancer cells continued. Buoyed by the notion that the cancer could be operable, and getting input from friends who had undergone prostatectomy, Perry found another center that could do the scan sooner, and at which robotic surgery on the prostate was performed. He also began looking for other urologic surgeons in New York in case the Prostascint scan was positive and the guy we had visited wouldn't operate.

A good friend who had undergone prostatectomy for benign enlargement told Perry that he would ask his son's father-in-law, the head of urologic surgery at Mayo Clinic, for recommendations. A day later we were in telephone conversation with the in-law, who opined that the case was operable in good hands and that there were four urologic surgeons he could wholeheartedly recommend: himself, but he was retired from active practice, the man he trained at Mayo, and two at the famous cancer hospital, one of whom now functioned in a mostly administrative capacity.

Mention of the surgeon who had recommended Prostascint scan was met with distinctly unfavorable noises. Likewise the response to the option of robotic surgery. The first available appointment with the famous cancer hospital surgeon in active practice was more than a month off, but the man at Mayo called the next day and within 24 hours he had scheduled Perry for radical prostatectomy with extensive lymph node dissection, the date calendared being one day before his birthday. He had no use or need for the Prostascint scan.

We canceled the scan, canceled the appointments with the Prostacint and robotics-leaning surgeons, and booked a flight to Rochester.

The following day the assistant of the surgeon at the famous cancer hospital called to say that the surgeon had been persuaded by the referral letter I had written and could see Perry within days. Furthermore, he had concluded that surgery was indicated, that outcomes were better than with radiation, that he was not a fan of hormonal therapy, and that he could operate within the week. Everyone, including the Mayo surgeon, said Perry was in the best hands.

We canceled Mayo, eating the airfare, canceled the return visit and surgery scheduled at the other hospital.

Hardly the same circumstance but reminiscent of a movie scene where the wife finds out her husband (George Segal) had arranged a romantic seaside vacation. She makes elaborate arrangements for her parents and children, thinking the reservations are for her, when in fact they're for George's new-found paramour. When George discovers this he tells the travel agent to cancel the flights! Cancel the hotel! Cancel everything!

In his brief meeting with me while Perry was taken to recovery the surgeon's remarks were cast with decided optimism; resectable lesion, good surgical planes, yes there was a positive node on frozen section but he got everything, no reason to expect anything other than what he expected. When I asked if there was much blood loss, he said that Perry bled as if he were taking aspirin, which he was not.

A most compliant patient, he had faithfully adhered to the proscription against use of aspirin in the days before surgery. My husband was a man who, scheduled to return for regular teeth cleaning at three month intervals, did so even when the appointment fell on the day before his prostate surgery - yes, he played tennis and had his teeth cleaned, joking that it was either a useless waste of money if he didn't survive the operation or a show of supreme optimism should it come up roses.

I shared, in this post-surgery meeting, my husband's preoperative desire not to mention his unexplained bleeding tendency that had periodically surfaced after tooth extraction and minor traumas. I also shared Perry's statement that "I'd rather bleed out on the table than suffer the agony of death from metastatic cancer that my father and Ronnie did." This was the only outward acknowledgement he made of the seriousness of his disease. The surgeon smiled, said there was no coagulation abnormality in the pre-op workup, and bleeding was not anything he couldn't handle. Maybe not, but pre-op hemoglobin was 17 and post-op it was 8.9 which, with a still functioning bone marrow, was able to soon return to normal.

Chapter 6

FALSE OPTIMISM

The final pathology was less rosy: a nasty cancer with Gleason 9+ score, involvement of both seminal vesicles, perineural invasion, two positive local nodes (although no evidence of cancer in a dozen resected inguinal nodes on each side), and a positive margin at the bladder neck, which some considered a more advanced stage. In the next few days I found a number of publications, mostly by the famous cancer hospital urologic surgeons, questioning whether positive margins warranted a more advanced classification that had prognostic significance.

The surgeon must have had faith in his own skills, announcing at the post-op visit in February that the PSA drawn that day would likely be less than 1. Convinced of his own optimism, he scheduled Perry for follow up return in June.

In an urgent call the following day the surgeon's assistant said the PSA was 11 and Perry should see an oncologist as soon as possible, suggesting three names from which I picked the woman, based on her publications and investigative record. Her next available appointment was one month later. I asked the surgeon to personally intervene to get a sooner appointment, which was promptly followed by a call from the oncologist's assistant offering a time in the upcoming week and saying that the doctor would be coming to the clinic expressly to see Perry.

The new appointment fell on the very day we had tickets to fly to Florida for a brief respite. We took the appointment and changedthe tickets - with a steep price penalty.

Chapter 7

THE ONCOLOGIST PRONOUNCES

The oncologist was more attractive in her website picture than in person. Small in stature, with a forced smile of geniality, she had a hard face that was accentuated by long straight bangs hanging into her eyes. To her credit, she did not keep us waiting long. Sweeping into the examining room, she promptly ordered us where to sit, insisting that we be side-by-side and sidewise to her desk so that she could look directly at both of us while talking. She commenced a didactic presentation on what the elevated PSA level represented. She said the increase in PSA was often seen, it could be spurious - not to worry - she had many patients like this and cited one - now going on fifteen years - with findings just the same.

Expounding further on the elevated PSA, she called it a "biochemical failure", which registered with me as inaccurate since the term is usually employed for a rise in PSA after a period of low to undetectable levels. This was certainly not the case with Perry, whose pre-op PSA was 15 and was close to that in the first measurement after surgery.

Then she launched into a long dissertation on prostate cancer, interspersed with self-congratulatory accolades about her experience and expertise. Winding up her discourse, she said that Perry could choose between watching and waiting, taking an anti-androgen that she liked to use off-label, or entering a Phase 2 clinical trial with Avastin, a drug that blocks a growth factor called VEGF. Her recommendation of the latter agent was puzzling, given that studies had shown that this agent did not prolong survival in patients with prostate cancer. I wondered if she received compensation for enrolling patients in additional clinical trials of the drug.

I noticed little bits of spittle at the corners of her mouth when she talked, thereafter privately referring to her as Dr. Slobber. Her lengthy but simplified explanation of the rationale behind each approach was delivered with carefully honed authoritarianism. No questions were allowed during her discourse that included, in reference to anti-androgens, the comment "men really do think with their gizmo." I found it hard to believe that a woman physician whose specialty was a cancer occurring only in men would gratuitously make such an offensively demeaning sexist comment.

She then told Perry to get on the examination table, performed the briefest of physical exams in which she cursorily palpated his neck - presumably for distant nodes - completely missed his premature ventricular contractions, and deferred the rectal exam with the quip "I'll spare you the indignity." She ordered some tests and abruptly left the room.

After my husband's death, when I got access to his medical records, I discovered that her notes from this first visit were entirely different from what actually transpired, as was the case for every other encounter with Dr. Slobber as well as with most other members of the hospital's medical oncology prostate cancer team.

Over the ensuing two years of Perry's life, we both came to realize that Dr. Slobber regularly practiced operation ostrich, holding forth with an unmistakable attitude that hers was the true explanation and rejecting any dialogue as opinionated, biased and uninformed. Unable to abide a truth she found disagreeable, she simply denied it, masterfully turning the slightest interjection after her pronouncements into an expression of little more than anger and/or ignorance on the part of the questioner.

Experience has provided an appreciation that an attending physician may be encased in a fragile self-protective membrane of insecurity and ego, easily ruptured by requests for information that are perceived as questioning competency. To question is to accuse. To ask for information is a challenge. Not to do so could violate one's own Hippocratic Oath as a physician. . Experience has also imbued an awareness of Murphy's Law that seems to perversely prevail for physicians and close relatives of physicians who encounter the medical system. Surgical mishaps, post-operative complications, iatrogenic infections, toxic drug effects, and all manner of rare and not-so-rare problems will abound. Following simple cholecystectomy, one professional colleague developed abdominal adhesions and bowel obstruction, requiring surgery to lyse the adhesions. Post-operatively, he had a pulmonary embolus. Anti-coagulated, he bled internally and developed a retroperitoneal hematoma that required surgical evacuation. Following this procedure, he developed acute renal failure, necessitating dialysis. When he returned to work some months after the initial surgery, he would wistfully and resignedly respond to sympathetic expressions about his troubled course: "These things happen". Alas and indeed, they do. A friend and neighbor who had successful surgery for a malignancy in the eye, entered the hospital about a year thereafter for a minor procedure, developed a hospital-acquired bacterial infection with colonization and destruction of his aortic valve which was removed and replaced with a porcine valve that became infected, giving rise to septicemia and multiple organ failure, and he died. Not fair. A good man.

In truth Dr. Slobber had misjudged his disease at the first encounter, a fact that became obvious at the return visit when the test results were in. The PSA was over 13, the CAT and bone scans showed metastatic disease. Dr. Slobber only offered a small confession:

"I'm surprised." This was the crumb from the doctor who 10 days earlier had told Perry he'd be "just fine" with a certitude and self-confidence that buoyed us in good spirits to enjoy a few days of sun in Florida.

She had been so wrong. How I could I have confidence in her self-proclaimed clinical acumen? I was acutely depressed but not surprised. If she remembered her comforting discourse at the first visit, it was an embarrassment to her and I certainly was not going to mention it. With time, I learned that she said a lot of things for which she had selective memory deficits, and also had a fair degree of inattentiveness until after the fact. I had a clear sense that she didn't cotton to me; as a woman, or as a physician, or both. I sat there mute - as do so many patients and relatives, and for the same reason: we are afraid to comment or question lest it be interpreted as an attack on the doctor's authority or expertise, which could prompt an expression of resentment by giving less than optimum care to our loved ones. I entertained the thought that it might be in Perry's best interest if I didn't accompany him on future visits.

I recalled listening to her describe the course of treatment predicated by the flourish - "Can I put it into remission? Absolutely!" I had a flashing recollection of Alec Baldwin in the movie *Malice* retorting to a lawyer's question - '*How does it feel playing god*' with '*I don't play, I am god*!'.

Chapter 8

OTHER OPTIONS

We got a callback from a radiation therapist on staff at the famous cancer hospital who we had contacted previously, offering an early March appointment. He had treated Stage 4 Gleason 8 prostate cancer in someone we knew, who was seven years without recurrence. There was nothing to lose, aside from the opprobrium of Dr. Slobber, from whom we did not request permission This radiation therapist, who was also a yarmulke-wearer, delivered his opinion in confidence-inspiring manner and tone - namely that radiation was not indicated, the disease was systemic, and the consequences of radiation to the surgical site could negatively impact continence and have other undesirable side-effects. He recommended anti-androgen therapy and then, when necessary, chemotherapy, saying that we could discuss which agents with Dr. Slobber. To my comment that she might not be amenable to such discussions, he responded, "I know exactly what you mean, enough said." He none too subtly validated my initial impressions of her omniscient delusions.

The descriptive details, along with a true grasp of the meaning of systemic disease, did not particularly register with Perry – but what he heard and what he understood was that, unlike our acquaintance, his prostate cancer could not be cured with radiation, and that he was dependent on the experience and judgment of Dr. Slobber, who he didn't like any better than I, but whose wisdom he was terrified of questioning.

Chapter 9

A SEARCH FOR MEANING

About a month after Perry commenced a regimen consisting of two drugs to block testosterone production, I accompanied him to one of the series of evening seminars he was attending on Judaism and existentialism. Invigorated by a contemplation of the mortality he faced, he was searching, and expressed a burgeoning interest in topics related to rabbinical teachings and religious observance. He was not without a solid foundation in such matters, instilled in his youth, during which he internalized the principle of Tikkun Olam – *Repairing the world*. He had shared with me that as a child he had secretly harbored the notion that he could be one of the mythical last of the just, but relinquished this idea when he was 11 and lost his temper while babysitting his sister after she had made a big mess in her diaper. From this incident he concluded that he was unworthy.

I was more inclined to historicity and etiology of the Bible than faith and observance, but I wanted to explore what Perry wanted to explore. He greatly admired Neil Gillman, the discussion leader that evening, a noted theologian and emeritus professor of the Jewish Theological Seminary. Neil opened the seminar by relating his own recent diagnosis of a malignancy in the parotid gland. He uncomplainingly noted his bad luck that his tumor was not one of the 75% of parotid gland tumors that are benign - adding quickly that he wasn't a statistic. *"This is me, my cancer,"* he said, going on to describe his experience of an intense loneliness after the surgery. I was mistaken in thinking that these remarks would resonate with Perry, who robustly disagreed, saying that the statistics of one's cancer are applicable and extremely meaningful in setting the probabilities of survival. Nevertheless, he came away from the seminar inspired, his faith bolstered. Neil Gillman outlived Perry by five years, cause of death in his obituary was ascribed to cancer.

Some months after that theological discussion, what Neil had to say about his subsequent course resonated with us both, even if for different reasons. Readmitted to the hospital for a wound infection, Neil developed a severe allergic reaction to the antibiotics from which he recovered sufficiently to be discharged, only to fall soon thereafter while carefully making his way along Broadway, requiring readmission for his injuries. But he found humor in the situation, relating how he kept telling the crowd that hovered on the pavement around him that he didn't have a stroke, he simply fell and, although his hip was intact, couldn't get up. Perry remembered these things when he, too, experienced side effects of drugs, and had his own fall upon an icy pavement. For me, Neil's tale exemplified the notion of "these things happen".

Chapter 10

SIDE EFFECTS

Within a week of starting the anti-androgen drug casodex Perry began itching and developed a steadily worsening eruption of red papules over his torso and limbs that he tried to alleviate with benadryl, to little avail. An old adage from my medical training says: *if you hear hooves on the bridge you don't think of zebras*. This was clearly an allergic reaction to the only new medication to which he had been introduced. This simple deduction was apparently beyond the ken of Dr. Slobber, who referred him, via her assistant, to a dermatologist who biopsied one of the papules which - surprise surprise - showed an inflammatory cell infiltration of an allergic response. The dermatologist also biopsied two raised spots of different character about which Perry asked, one on the scalp which showed actinic keratosis – a benign lesion that sometimes turns malignant - and another at the temple which showed squamous cell carcinoma in situ (no invasion seen on pathology and totally excised in the biopsy), prompting the dermatologist to refer him to another dermatologist. Talk about overspecialization. And the next week he had to have a root canal. Talk about when it rains it pours.

The rash responded to prednisone but meanwhile Perry began complaining of discomfort in both groins. I was watching him like a proverbial hawk, questioned him in detail about the nature of the pain, and scurried to re-read the bone scan report to find out exactly where those metastatic foci were located, wildly but silently asking if this could be bone pain. The CAT scan had shown walled off lymphatic accumulations on both sides, not alarming, and provided a comforting explanation for both the discomfort and a noted stiffness in walking and slowing of his ability to get around on the tennis court, all of which improved as time went by, as an aftermath of surgery. The PSA was a wonderful 0.19 six weeks after start of the anti-androgen program, evidence that it was working. At the 12 weeks visit, the day of the second injection of Lupron – the companion anti-androgen in his course of treatment - the PSA was 0.55, an upward blip that I silently registered with concern. Perry questioned Dr. Slobber, who pooh-poohed it.

Chapter 11

INTERCURRENT PROBLEMS - DR. SOUP APPEARS

Perry was watching his nightly dose of Fox news the evening after the second dose of Lupron when he suddenly had a shaking chill with a slight fever, some gastrointestinal upset and a diffuse sense of unwellness. He couldn't describe exactly what he felt, simply said that he just knew *something wasn't right.* I thought he might be having a drug reaction or had been exposed to a contaminated injection of the Lupron. The next day he was worse. We went to urgent care at the hospital. The physician who examined him thought it could be a urinary tract infection and after a phone consultation with Dr. Slobber decided to admit him. Little comfort that the urine was sterile since radiographic studies showed a partial bowel obstruction, presumably due to adhesions and, like the lymphoceles, another surgical aftermath. Those lymphoceles were benign, but in retrospect reflected the vigor of the surgeon's hands, which I remembered were quite large, in manipulating the operative field, entered retropubically, not through the abdominal cavity.

The bowel obstruction responded to symptomatic treatment, but the CAT scan, which confirmed the obstruction, also showed increased number and size of bony metastases in the pelvis and elsewhere, with a lytic lesion spanning the width of one side of the pubic bone. The attending oncologist, soon to be nicknamed Dr. Soup, definitively opined that the bowel obstruction had nothing to do with his cancer and pooh-poohed the increase in skeletal metastases, saying that it was not in a weight-bearing bone. He was unperturbed by the 3 gram drop in hemoglobin that had occurred in less than a week after the last clinic visit, and proclaimed that the PSA had shown a straight downward course, failing to notice that the PSA was clearly rising with an admission value of 5.5. His ignorance of the disease history and lack of clinical acumen were breathtaking.

A year later, during my husband's last two weeks at the famous cancer hospital, Dr. Soup was again the inpatient attending. He greeted Perry on morning rounds: "Nice to meet you." Perry immediately recognized him and marked his inattentiveness by calling him out with a calmly-delivered: "We have met before."

I dubbed the man Dr. Soup because his limited capacity could do little more than homogenize patients into one unidentifiable mixture and his name rhymed with the famous brand.

Chapter 12

RELAPSE

Dr. Slobber did note the elevated PSA, which was over 20 at the next outpatient visit, and discontinued the casodex, saying that it might no longer be effective – *how could she doubt the evidence?* She added that sometimes there can be a period of remission when casodex is stopped, but she would wait to see what the next CAT and bone scans showed. The scans predictably confirmed multiple new bony metastasis, some with lytic components, in the thoracic spine and in the ribs that were not noted in previous scans, new lesions in right femur, and a growing lytic lesion in the left pubic bone. Inexplicably, her notes read: "Bone scan suggests improvement." She ordered a PET scan to "better see what's going on." Pending that, she said if the PSA started to rise - *which it already had* - she would consider either docetaxel or ketoconazole, and wrote in her notes: "The physician wife is disinclined to ketoconazole, wants abiraterone or docetaxel, but abiraterone cannot be given unless patient has treatment failure to chemotherapy and docetaxel should be held in reserve."

Again unsurprisingly, the PET scan showed numerous glucose avid mixed lytic/sclerotic metastasis including the clavicle, 5th and 7th thoracic vertebral bodies, right 6th rib, sacral promontory, right iliac bone, pelvic soft tissue and around the vesico-urethral anastomosis, all unequivocally indicating disease progression. Yet I was stunned to find that she again wrote in her notes: "The patient has had mixed response on his scans" and told us the same. The next PSA was over 80. She pushed ketoconazole, justifying herself in her notes with the following entry:

"I do not feel that chemotherapy is emergent at this time. I have elected instead to go forward with ketoconazole (Nizoral). The patient's wife is a retired endocrinologist who has been involved with aminoglutethimide and has an understanding of adrenal pathways. She was concerned that he would become adrenal insufficient and I explained to her that this was unlikely at the dose given. We also discussed the rationale for abiraterone for which I will attempt to obtain a prescription at some point. He and his wife are aware of the rationale for changing to chemotherapy, including but not limited to rapid PSA rises and short doubling time, failure to thrive, or widespread symptomatic disease for which chemotherapy would likely spare the marrow in lieu of radiation. We discussed side effects of Nizoral including fatigue, dry skin, elevated liver function tests, nausea/vomiting. Patient will be going with wife for 3-day trip to tennis camp."

Chapter 13

DR. SLOBBER ARROGANTLY PREVAILS

Early in my career, intrigued by a report of adrenal insufficiency in patients taking the anti-convulsant aminoglutethimide, I discovered the mechanism of action responsible for its anti-adrenal effects which, after this and other reports, were therapeutically exploited in the old days in patients with breast and prostate cancer. I suppose she googled my publications to learn this, I didn't query, but I did register my dislike of ketoconazole. Disdaining my unenthusiastic comment, Dr. Slobber pronounced that she knew best and wrote a prescription for ketoconazole, a drug with inhibitory effects on the production of steroids, a class of substances produced by the adrenal cortex and the testes to which both cortisol and testosterone belong. Poisonous to fungi, when administered systemically to people, it has a host of gastrointestinal and other side effects, including blocking adequate production of cortisol by the adrenal gland.

A week or so after starting the drug, Perry developed an allergic swelling, discomfort and purplish discoloration of the inside lining of the lips which intensified as days passed. He called Dr. Slobber's office and was triaged by the physician's assistant who said she would check with the doctor. She called back late that afternoon to convey the opinion from on high: "Don't eat so many purple grapes." *What impressive clinical acumen without examining the oral mucosa!* And need I add, Perry never ate purple grapes, he didn't like the seeds. Without subsequent query if the swelling and discoloration had subsided, she continued the schedule of increasing dosage in the weeks that followed, opining that supplemental steroids were not necessary at these dosages, but it became very clear within a month that they were.

Board certified in internal medicine and the subspecialty of endocrinology and metabolism, I ought to recognize adrenal insufficiency when I see it. Late that summer, when we were on vacation in Italy, I did. I found Perry weak and dizzy in the hot Tuscan sun, sitting at a little table in the plaza of San Gimignano, head down on crossed arms, sweating profusely, and pulse racing. I looked frantically for a pharmacy in the little square, but finding none I ran for lemonade, water, salt, which I forced him to down. His appearance and heart rate improved over the next hour, but his appetite remained abysmal and his physical tolerance low for the rest of the trip.

Chapter 14

WHEN IT RAINS IT POURS

Not long after returning from Italy, Perry found me brushing my teeth as he emerged from the shower and asked - "what's this?" - pointing to a very large lump in his groin. It was firm, not hard, looked and felt like a hernia, but I wasn't sure that I could reduce it, meaning that I couldn't push it back into the abdomen, and of course the possibility of a giant metastatic mass crossed my alarmist mind. I called the single attending physician who had exhibited compassion and concern during the previous hospitalization for the bowel obstruction; the one physician who had personally contacted me after reviewing the CAT scan to tell me that there was no evidence of peritoneal carcinomatosis. She was a general surgeon who had seen Perry to evaluate if need be for surgical intervention, and she was the only physician who had offered her cell phone number.

Graciously, she saw him that afternoon, confirmed the hernia, advised surgery, and scheduled the operation as soon as possible. Perry felt obliged to notify Dr. Slobber, also posing my question about need for supplemental cortisol, which she pooh-poohed, saying his adrenals were just fine. Fortunately, the surgeon followed the advice of the internist and anesthesiologist who were consulted for medical clearance for surgery and prescribed the standard pre-op cortisol recommended for people with compromised adrenal function. Notwithstanding, as they prepared to discharge him from the recovery room, I found his pulse escalated to 150 when he stood and suggested a bit more fluid and a bit more time. The surgeon commented that his tissue was very fragile, but I was relieved that he tolerated the surgery and that it was, after all, just a hernia and not a cancerous mass.

Chapter 15

RESPITE

A few weeks later, the request for third party coverage for treatment with abiraterone, a recently approved inhibitor of testosterone production, was allowed. The PSA was over 80, the ill-advised ketoconazole, having been completely ineffective, was discontinued. There was a glorious response to abiraterone with the PSA nadiring to less than one, and on the high of that lab result we went to Puerto Rico for a few days of sun and some tennis. Perry played with excellent strokes but did not go after those cross-court balls that, with his long legs, he had always managed to get. He made an appointment at the hotel spa for a facial and figuring that it would be accompanied by a neck massage and worried about cervical spine lesions, I quietly told the personnel to omit it.

Chapter 16

SETBACK

About a month after return from Puerto Rico, Perry slipped and fell backward on an icy sidewalk. He lay there a few moments before rising and, like Neil Gilman, insisted he was okay and that he didn't need anything, he would wait for his next clinic appointment.

Alas, the PSA was 16 at that visit. Dr. Slobber abruptly discontinued the abiraterone, telling Perry not to worry, there were other agents. Eschewing docetaxel, the standard chemotherapy for castration resistant prostate cancer, she promoted enrollment in various clinical trials, writing down the names and drawing incomprehensible circles and arrows. Her notes from that visit, summarizing Perry's course since his initial visit the previous year read:

"The patient had a brief response to hormonal therapy. I spent one hour with patient and physician wife discussing treatment options. I have strongly encouraged them to look to investigational trials with biological agents that may impact on the biology of the cancer. His physician wife was adamantly against his being treated with biological agents, saying they could be associated with significant side effects. I gently corrected her and indicated that this has not been the case and that we have had much success with a variety of different biologic agents that may impact very effectively on the tumor. Wife and patient disinclined to go forward with docetaxel. Wife expressed interest in the radium 223 agent Alpharadin which is unavailable at this time. I reviewed in detail rational and associated side effects of various investigational protocols including PSMA-directed autologous T-cells, IMC-A12 and temsirolimus, ARN-509, and Enzon's EZN-4176 as well as standard docetaxel. At this time patient's wife is leaning toward ARN-509. He will be contacted once ARN-509, her first choice, becomes available which should be within next 10 days."

Chapter 17

PREVARICATIONS AND OBFUSCATIONS

As Dr. Slobber's notes verified, I was with him at that visit in late February. And I have a clear recollection of what transpired. After reading her notes my reaction was *liar liar pants on fire!*

The "response to hormonal therapy" was not quite accurate. There had been a brief biochemical response reflected in the PSA level, but the blossoming metastatic lesions and accelerated disease progression were documented on multiple imaging studies. I was totally inclined to docetaxel and so said. She had, in fact, previously proposed alpha radon (Radium 223) in combination with docetaxel as her first choice, subsequently negating that approach at the next visit, saying that protocol was on hold due to depression of white cells accompanied with fever. I had expressed concern about biological agents in view of Perry's history of allergic response, noting that he had once experienced an anaphylactic reaction with laryngeal edema, etiology unknown but possibly related to a seasonal allergy and that he had anti-thyroid antibodies, a marker of propensity to immune reaction.

"What is your preference?" I had asked. She leaned forward or sat back, I can't remember, but her look of patronizing dominance is etched in my memory. "There are three good options," she said and proceeded to lay them out. The first was transfusion of the patient's own T-cells transfected with a viral vector expressing prostate membrane-specific antigen to hone in on prostate cancer cells. The second was an antibody directed against the insulin-like growth factor receptor coupled with an inhibitor of the mTOR cell signaling pathway. The third was the androgen receptor inhibitor known as ARN. The first was her own devise. She was conducting a Phase 1 trial in which she was eager to enroll patients; there had been no evidence to date of efficacy in people, she had tried it in exactly four patients, one progressed and the other three were promising but "too early to tell." *And she wanted my husband to consent to this?*

This from the woman who had made disparaging clucking noises about Provenge, an immunotherapeutic approach in which the patient's own white blood cells are coupled to a prostate antigen and then infused into the patient, opining that the reported 3-4 months increased survival was a fluke, the series too small to be meaningful. Her detailed review of IMC-A12 (a monoclonal antibody) given with the anti-cancer drug temsirolimus consisted of drawing a bunch of circles with various arrows that Perry found unfathomable. Likewise her half-sentence allusion to EZN-4176, an androgen blocker in a phase 1 study to merely assess safety, was hardly illuminating. Perry was, however, familiar with the concept of decreasing effects of testosterone, and was instinctively inclined to ARN-509, a new androgen receptor blocker in Phase 2 studies. Dr Slobber reinforced his inclination with her statement, in no uncertain terms that "This is my first choice, it is the perfect treatment, this is the drug for you. We have to wait six weeks for abiraterone to clear your system, and then we can start." Perry asked again about docetaxel which Dr. Slobber again eschewed. She wanted another CAT and bone scan before his next visit, scheduled for about six weeks later.

Six weeks with no treatment, while his disease galloped onward, did not faze her.

Chapter 18

WAITING

In early March, awaiting the scan reports at the next scheduled visit with Dr. Slobber, we went to the national AIPAC shebang in Washington. We had been attending it together for several consecutive years, and Perry was indefatigable in his attentiveness in the sessions and gregariousness in the social milieu. But that year he was restless in his seat, not complaining, but registering clear signs of an inability to sustain a comfortable position. He was between therapies, purportedly waiting for the abiraterone to clear from his system and start the next program, without which progression of his disease was accelerating. The root of his discomfort no doubt stemmed from bony metastases, but he persevered at the sessions and did not hesitate in pre-registering for the next year's conference. It was an article of faith, not a desire to take advantage of the early bird discount, and I did nothing to dissuade him, ardently hoping he'd live to attend.

He did not, but what great satisfaction he would have had to know that one of our sons attended in his stead, and then signed up to attend the following year.

The scans showed collapse of the 7th thoracic vertebra, along with widespread metastases throughout the spine and in the pelvis, and multiple new lesions in both long bones of the arms and legs. An MRI a couple days later confirmed the vertebral body collapse and evidence of invasion in the marrow of the 8th vertebral body. The collapsed vertebra likely stemmed from acute injury of diseased bone consequent to his fall, about which he had been stoic. The PSA had risen, the alkaline phosphatase, which in part reflected the widespread bony metastasis but a substantial part of which probably arose from the vertebral collapse, was off the chart. Even Dr. Slobber recognized that these were not "let's wait and see" findings, and that absent the discontinued abiraterone or indeed other therapy, the disease was indeed galloping. Yet she wanted a PET scan "to be sure," which of course affirmed the widespread disease. She referred him to a neurosurgeon to undertake a procedure to stabilize the thoracic spine.

We appreciated the neurosurgeon's frankness in stating that he would not have the procedure if he were in Perry's shoes, although, to my chagrin, I subsequently learned that his consultative report (electronically signed) located the collapse in the wrong thoracic vertebra.

Chapter 19

HIDDEN EVIL

It was not until some months after my husband's death that I discovered, in reviewing his medical records, the true perniciousness of electronic signatures as well as the major ethical and legal problems inherent therein. Dr. Slobber's notes were hand-written – and thus accurately quoted herein – but most often reports are composed by house officers in computerized entries. The attending physician merely clicks a box attesting that he or she has personally reviewed and agrees with everything described; giving rise to an indelibility of errors and fabrications that can punctuate reports of a patient encounter or a procedure that is perpetuated without question.

This evil came home to roost when I read the neurosurgeon's note describing collapse of the wrong vertebra. Equally horrifying, I also read electronically signed descriptions of full explanation of the risks of – *and my concurrence with* – treatment proposed by physicians responsible for my husband's care whom *I had never met* and with whom *discussion was nonexistent*.

Chapter 20

CHANGE OF COURSE

Eagerly anticipating commencement of the recommended drug, Perry was flabbergasted at the next visit when, completely nonplussed, Dr. Slobber announced that he could not get ARN-509 because "they changed the protocol, patients who had received ketoconazole were not eligible for that drug."

Did she deliberately lie? Was this merely another example of her inattentiveness, of which there were and continued to be multiple examples?

The fact was that the protocol, filed with the FDA, indicated that prior treatment with ketoconazole was an absolute exclusion criterion, and that there had been no subsequent protocol change, of which the FDA must be notified. That Perry had a dated hard copy of the protocol, and that the government site had posted the original protocol as well as a record of any changes, had little impact on her confidence that he would swallow her bold-faced lie.

He burst into tears, stripped of his hope that he would be given this new therapy, touted so grandly by his oncologist Dr. Slobber, the person in whom he had placed his future. Perhaps she thought the written protocol details were beyond him, or that he was unfamiliar with clinical trials.gov, but surely, she did not think such was beyond his wife, who stifled voicing any awareness to the contrary. Patting his knee, Dr. Slobber opined that his life "did not depend on ARN." When asked again about Alpharadin, which she had recommended on previous visits, and was subsequently shown to increase survival, Dr. Slobber waved it off with the comment "it's just for bone pain, doesn't attack cancer cells" and anyway the trial was "on hold because some neutropenia had been noted, probably innocuous but sometimes accompanying febrile episodes."

The PSA was further elevated and Perry was crushed at the prospect of being without treatment. He was reliant on Dr. Slobber's judgment and had faith in her strong recommendation of ARN. His despair deepened as she again marched into a recitation of initials and numbers of various available trials and acronyms of the respective agents. She kept talking and he couldn't make sense of anything she said. She commented that he probably wouldn't have responded long-term to ARN and wrote in her notes that I asked about a PI3K inhibitor, which she said was not available, which meant that she was not participating in the sponsor's clinical trials. And absent that, docetaxel could be indicated but she didn't like to use it until all else failed. Perry was torn about making the right decision. She had given him more than half a dozen informed consent packages detailing protocols for the various investigational agents she had mentioned, with instructions to read them and decide.

Overwhelmed, Perry brought them home, attempted to make some sense of them, but was left bewildered and bereft. He had told her in no uncertain terms that her little drawings of overlapping circles and mumblings about pathways, with pathway number one affecting pathway number two, were entirely unfathomable and bewildering and politely stated that he needed to discuss with me. He also said he didn't know how anyone could decide.

Chapter 21

BADGERING

He returned a week later, alone. Dr. Slobber's entry indicated it was a treatment decision visit, that they again talked about phase 1/2 trials and that the wife, who was uncomfortable with such, was not present, prompting the presence of a nurse, presumably as a witness. Perry had brought a list of questions about docetaxel versus the other treatments, looking for specific answers regarding relative risk/benefit in relation to side effects that he could understand, taking notes of her responses.

Perry: "What is the benefit of docetaxel?"
Dr. Slobber: "Destroys cancer cells, but not every one, and not with certainty, and duration of benefit is limited."
Perry: "What are the specific reasons you don't like giving docetaxel?"
Dr. Slobber: "I like to avoid it until it's really needed. I like to save it until there is bone pain."

How could she not register that this was exactly what he was experiencing, multiple bony lesions corroborated by the various scans?

She elaborated, saying that standard chemo can be toxic and not all patients respond and "we want to change the environment of the cancer and prevent tumor growth or cause tumor shrinking."

Perry: "What is the benefit of IMC-A12 plus temsirolimus?"
Dr. Slobber: "It shrinks cancer cells."
Perry: "How does it do this?"
Dr. Slobber: no response.

Perry: "How many people have received IMC-temsirolimus?"
Dr. Slobber: "I'll look it up."
Perry: "Is this treatment contraindicated if tumor growth continues?"
Dr. Slobber: shrugs.

Perry tried another tack, asking what the test criterion is regarding whether the treatment is attacking cancer cells and if there is a basis for believing that the chance of preventing tumor growth or shrinking tumor size is greater than one in two.
Dr. Slobber: "I have a good gestalt about this."
He phrased the question another way, asking has this been observed in animals or people, and are there publications supporting this.
Dr. Slobber: "There seems to be synergism. I don't have any publications handy, the benefit is uncertain, cancer cells may continue attacking bone, multiply and spread, duration of benefit is limited, potential side effects are unknown. There is a chance that PSA will rise and/or cancer will grow with the experimental treatment, which we don't expect but has happened in earlier studies."
Perry: "Have there been allergic reactions of IMC-A12?"
Dr. Slobber: "No."

Her one word response contradicted specific mention of such in the list of side effects.

Perry: "What alternative do you recommend and why?"
Dr. Slobber: "There is no alternative."

Perry had found a press release on the internet about an IMC-A12 plus temsirolimus trial, provided by ImClone, the maker of the anti-IGF receptor monoclonal antibody. He appended this to his handwritten notes. Mention is made of preclinical studies and some phase 1 safety and pharmacokinetic profiles. He was being enrolled in a really early and small trial of an agent with scant and unproven benefit, with notice in the consent form that his choices if he did not take part in the study were: 1) treatment or care without being in a study, 2) taking part in another study, 3) getting no treatment. He suspected that the aversion to docetaxel hinged on Dr. Slobber's desire to enroll patients in the IMC-temsirolimus trial, for which she was compensated.

She dodged his question about the next treatment if IMC-temsirolimus did not suffice, merely noting that the informed consent says he can withdraw at any time, a comment that left him justifiably disturbed.

Between the lines and according to his own account later that day, he did get a fair dose of badgering about her wisdom and a statement that she would always consider investigational approach for her own family member, one could always turn later to docetaxel or, even better, sign up for her own phase 1 T-cell trial. Her recorded entry said:
"The patient became tearful due to the overwhelming nature of the discussion and to the previous conversation in the wife's presence when she was unable to satisfy her concerns," then contradicting herself, continues: "He indicated he did not sense the latter at all and was very comfortable with what was ongoing."

I did not know of these notes at the time, but Perry's description of the interaction during the visit was starkly different. He had indeed become tearful, he told me, but this had little to do with conversations of the previous visit. He was acutely stripped of confidence in Dr. Slobber's pronouncements, his questions were whitewashed with platitudes, and he said he felt completely cowered. Admonishing him for not wanting to participate in her Phase 1 trial, she pushed for IMC-temsirolimus, and told him to come back with the executed consent form.

What does a man, battling his own mortality, do when his oncologist, an authority in the very disease threatening his life badgers, berates, belittles, scolds and threatens him?

Chapter 22

ACQUIESCENCE

After his death I discovered Perry's handwritten notes scattered in his file drawers. Pondering his disease, symptoms and treatment, they were heartbreaking to read. He looked for explanations as he recognized his downhill course, recorded his fear and distrust of Dr. Slobber, her continuous hedging and bold statements like "ARN is the drug for you." He simply wanted comprehensible answers to his specific questions of why and what was happening. He acknowledged being dependent on her, a dependency I suspect she cultivated.

At my husband's request and unbeknownst to Dr. Slobber, I consulted with the prostate cancer specialist at another institution whose advice we had sought the previous summer and whose opinion I respected. At that time the PSA was rising and the scans had shown evidence of increased number and size of skeletal metastases. Dr. Slobber had discontinued the casodex and wanted to start ketoconazole.

The specialist had suggested waiting a couple of weeks to see if the PSA remained stable or continued rising. If the latter occurred, he advised starting an androgen receptor blocker with docetaxel.

At this second consultation, he unequivocally stated that Perry was overdue for docetaxel, disagreeing with Dr Slobber that docetaxel was "the end of the line", there were other agents that could be used. He was not opposed to trying IMC-temsirolimus but firmly stated that it should be discontinued if there was no response after the first treatment cycle. We both liked the man, had respect for his judgment, appreciated his ready availability for consultation and talked about transferring Perry to his care. He was agreeable and suggested we discuss that possibility after the first cycle of the protocol.

Alas, when I spoke with him after that first cycle he had accepted a position at another institution in another city. Transferring Perry to his care was impossible.

So Perry consented to the IMC-temsirolimus protocol #09-117 under Dr. Slobber's continued care. The long list of side effects included serious allergic manifestations and life-threatening anaphylaxis that fortified my resolve to attend each treatment. Dr. Slobber sarcastically commented: "We will be so comforted you are there."

But he held off on signing the accompanying protocol #90-040 for tumor biopsies that were strictly for undefined research purposes. He had thoroughly read the protocol and thought its purpose - to collect blood and tissue samples that may help learn more about prostate cancer and its treatment - was noble, but he was troubled by several elements, such as drawing extra blood, repeated biopsies, the absence of a sunset clause, and the long list of institutions and people with whom information can and will be shared. This seemed to conflict with the sentence that followed stating that whatever emerged from the study was protected information. He pressed Dr. Slobber about the dichotomy, noting that some of those on the list may not be subject to privacy laws. Her response, memorialized in his hand-written notes, was that he could choose to withdraw from the study at any time, but consent is necessary to collect payment for the care received while on the study and to run the business of the hospital, an argument he found counterproductive.

Dr. Slobber's note however reads, "He has refused to sign #90-040 even though this was explained to him in detail." My husband had taken a small stand in the face of her badgering.

Chapter 23

FAILURE

The first treatment was in early April and required that the series of scans that had been done barely a week before be repeated as baseline, and again at regular intervals. These showed the multiple diffuse metastatic bony lesions, with no appreciable change compared to the previous scans. The report also recommended an area in the left pubic bone as suitable for biopsy, evidently reflecting instructions to identify such despite Perry's refusal to sign the informed consent for tumor biopsies. Just before administration of the treatment he was required to re-consent to the IMC-temsirolimus protocol because of a change in the side effect profile that newly included high blood sugar and increased fatigue.

Returning three weeks later for the second treatment, Perry reported that he had been throwing up and didn't feel hungry. His weight was down more than six pounds. The PSA at the first treatment had been 175 and was now 310. This stunning increase exactly met the proviso made by the now unavailable oncologist we had consulted that the protocol be discontinued and docetaxel be initiated. Perry asked Dr. Slobber if the treatment was working and if the protocol should be discontinued. She dismissed his questions and his symptoms with a wave of her hand: "It's too early to tell, stick with it." The next visit for the third dose was scheduled for three weeks later, repeat scans ordered to see "how well you are responding".

Contrary to Dr. Slobber's statement, there were alternatives, at least one of which we raised with her as soon as it became clear that IMC A12 temsirolimus did nothing to halt disease progression. The Mayo clinic had a couple of spectacular regressions of advanced prostate cancer using a new immunotherapeutic that was having success with malignant melanoma. A straw, but a hope, although one that couldn't be pursued long distance. Surely the famous cancer hospital could offer this approach. But efforts to avail Perry of it met with disdain and rejection, the chief objection being that they had no clinical trial, double blind or not.

Less than two years after his death, the famous cancer hospital doctors were quoted in the press on their innovative thrust using DNA profiling to identify patients whose cancers might respond to agents used for other malignancies, which they would be giving to patients with resistant disease and absent any clinical trial for their particular malignancy. In fact, one of the agents was exactly that which I had proposed to Dr. Slobber for my husband. They had his DNA profile, courtesy of sampling done under the rubric of "for research purposes" when he was enrolled in the anti-IGF antibody/temsirolimus trial, and for which he had given informed consent. Yes, the agent had awful side effects, but even in the famous cancer hospital doctors' hands, subsequent to Perry's death, it has shown benefit and prolongation of life.

One of the notes I found in Perry's drawer was dated five days before his scheduled return for the third treatment. He had listed under the heading Side Effects the problems he had been experiencing since the second dose: fatigue during the day, loss of appetite, loss of taste, vomiting and retching when he tried to eat, constant thirst at night, a lesion on his tongue, weight loss, new and lasting pain in the right leg. He brought the list to the clinic but it was moot. The PSA was over 650.

Dr. Slobber abruptly discontinued the IMC-temsirolimus protocol, patted his knee and told him not to worry. "I have the right drug for you," she assured him. She wrote the letters down to bring to me and sent him home with descriptive material and an informed consent for the Phase 3 clinical trial of the drug, a spin-off of yet another androgen blocker, MDV-3100 that had been submitted for FDA approval.

Chapter 24

MORE INATTENTIVENESS

Perry began having difficulty walking during the interim waiting for his next visit - at which he was supposed to start MDV-3100 - along with right hip pain and pain emanating down the back of his leg. Dr. Slobber watched him hobbling into the examining room and made the woefully inhuman comment: "Look at you, you look like an old Bobe." Not realizing that the masculine Yiddish term is Zaide.

Perry asked about his lab work, which he had accessed online; noting an alarming drop in hemoglobin, low platelets, and stark elevations in measurements reflecting bone disease and in the acid phosphatase of prostate origin. Dr. Slobber rose regally from her chair, her face expressionless, and left the room without a word, believing her incognizance of the lab results would go unnoticed. She returned a few moments later and carefully ensconced herself back in the power seat with a smug smile. She proceeded to admonish Perry that the nonsteroidal anti-inflammatory he had been taking for pain was affecting his blood counts. Of course she could hardly acknowledge that she had left the room to look at the lab report, which she should have looked at before entering the room in the first place.

Where was that superior clinical acumen that failed to recognize that the falling platelets and hemoglobin reflected progression of his disease, encroaching on the bone marrow.

She began a long erudite commentary, ascribing the significant decreases in hemoglobin and platelets to: 1) low testosterone from Lupron - *if that were so, why had it only recently started to fall? He had been on Lupron for more than a year*, 2) an outside chance of bone marrow involvement - *which it most likely was,* 3) the Motrin he was taking daily for pain - *unlikely as it inhibits platelet aggregation but only rarely depresses bone marrow and Perry had no evidence of bleeding.* "Stay away from ibuprofen," she said, "we like Aleve."

Perry held fast to his opinion that something was different and asked for radiographs. The hospital could not schedule an MRI of the spine for some time, so Dr. Slobber sent him to a local private facility, waving him away with: "I'll call your wife later with the results."

She called at dinner time to report there was "nothing more than a little degenerative arthritis" and prescribed opiates for pain.

But the radiologist misread the films. The final report stated that there were extensive metastatic lesions with compression of the nerve roots below the end of the spinal cord and compromise of the spinal canal at the 7th thoracic vertebra, although without evidence of cord compression. A day later an MRI of the hip at the hospital facility showed extraosseous extension from metastases in the right ilium and from left pelvic bone signifying invasion of the bone marrow, confirming that the low platelets and hemoglobin arose from bone marrow compromise and that the real reason for hip/buttock pain had been ignored, as was the developing cauda equina syndrome.

Chapter 25

THE WIFE

It gave me no pleasure that my every intuition from the first elevated PSA to the escalating disease on the CAT scans proved correct, and the pronouncements of Dr. Slobber in dismissing these findings as little concern were undeniably wrong. I cannot rid myself of the conviction that my husband's life was shortened by ill-timed and ill-advised interventions; lack of the appropriate measures administered with unrelenting inhumanity by physicians who not once reciprocated his trust with clear explanation or choice; who practiced a game of infantilization and dependency, shrouded in bureaucratization and marginalization of any question of their authoritative voice of experience.

Nor was Perry the only recipient of such calculated deception, as I learned one afternoon in the outpatient waiting room. I overheard a man on his cell phone recounting the gist of his visit with Dr. Slobber. "She said it's only a couple of spots, not very big, not to worry, I can treat it." He was describing the newly appeared lesions in his lungs, an ominous finding indicative of systemic soft tissue metastasis of his prostate cancer. I shuddered.

Doctors loathe dealing with other doctors that do not belong to their own tight circle of referral and acquaintance, fearful of penetration of the carefully constructed façade of self-assurance that requires unquestioning docility. There are recognizable patterns of behavior in physicians who perceive intelligent discussion as a challenge to their authority. Dr. Slobber was a walking poster child for this syndrome. But there were other members of the prostate cancer oncology team at the famous cancer hospital who were clearly in this club. And we were about to meet them as Perry's disease progressed.

I believe physicians are good people. They want to do the right thing. They are taught to save lives and treat disease. But there is now a new concept, employed by patients, families and physicians, described as *unwanted care*, also called by some *wrongful care*. This notion arises from the belief that if people were more fully informed they would not want available but arduous prolongation of life, they would opt against what would be presented to them as unnecessary suffering for no ostensible purpose, and presented with cold facts and statistics, they would choose to die simply, at home or in hospice.

I'm not talking about sustaining life with mechanical respiration or resuscitation after cardiac arrest from terminal incurable disease, or the very aged who at some point decide not to eat, concluding that, as the mother of a childhood friend colorfully put it in Polish - *"Enough is enough and even the pigs won't eat it."*

But I dispute the perspective offered in a recent New York Times essay by a medical resident who regretted an episode during his internship when he ardently advocated a novel intervention that had a reasonable chance of ameliorating a patient's advanced heart failure. The procedure was described as uneventful, but a "rare but known" postoperative complication disrupted her heart rhythm and precipitated cardiac arrest, which could not be reversed by resuscitative measures. With the hindsight of a couple more years of residency training, the essayist concluded that, in arguing for the procedure, he had acted out of an irrational and misplaced optimism, and he retrospectively accused the patient of similar false hope. The resident had persuaded himself that substituting prognostic truths for state-of-the art treatment better serves the patient, but how could he be so sure that this or any person afflicted with incurable disease would so readily concur. The woman knew it was a temporizing intervention, a palliative procedure offering not a cure but a hope of affording her more time, more life, and she consented to the procedure with that understanding.

Chapter 26

THE HUSBAND

Nor was my husband of that resident's persuasion. He wanted to live. He wanted every possible treatment until he wanted to die and he knew when that was without further information. He needed no "conversation," even less a cold discussion of his "goals" from a heartless social worker. He tolerated every intrusion from the army of physicians, house officers, physicians' assistants, nurses, and so-called patient advocates who abrogated every rule of compassionate care. My professional takeaway was that the latter were, in fact, physician advocates, consistently coloring every attempt at discussion with a steely "doctor knows best" that obfuscated intelligent discourse.

Three months before he died Perry asked me to make plans for Paris, first class with wheelchair accommodation, looking forward to again happily eating his way across France. After his death I found handwritten notes of other plans for the future, including reserving the house in the Poconos for our annual family winter vacation. He wanted more time, more life, and that desire sustained his will even though it did not halt the progression of his disease. He never complained over daily indignities, nor of his reduced, increasingly undignified state. He rarely gave voice to pain or suffering and never mentioned "death with dignity."

His body was in bad state, but he was mens sana and could have handled any discussion of his prognosis and options - but alas none was offered to him. What he got from the staff physician Dr. Soup, the man who failed to read my husband's chart a year earlier and was equally ignorant of anything subsequent, was a cold announcement that there was nothing for him but hospice care. His note in the hospital record from that day reads:

"In answer to a direct question from the patient about treatment, I told him that I advise either home or inpatient hospice. We discussed the nature of hospice and he seemed shocked that he was indeed hospice appropriate. I told him that many patients have improved quality of life and some live longer by avoiding therapy that is unlikely to benefit. I told him that another oncology team at another hospital would not accept him and he was not a candidate for rehab."

Chapter 27

MENS SANA

Incredibly, in his brief visit on in-patient rounds the next morning, Dr. Soup informed my husband that he was depressed and needed consultation with a psychiatrist. Astounded, Perry asked me what would prompt Dr. Soup to make such a recommendation - to insert himself into the most personal of arenas without cause or evidence of psychiatric disequilibrium. I too was dumbfounded and tried a bit of humor to divert his reaction to Dr. Soup's pronouncement. and assuage his distraught state. I reminded him of an incident the previous year with Perry's roommate, an Asian man. I heard a white-coated resident tell the patient that his doctors thought he was confused and asked for the psychiatry team to evaluate him. "I'm going to give you a little memory test," the resident explained. "I am going to say three words and I want you to repeat them - barn, horse, velvet." Silence from the patient. Again the instructions came, the last word drawn out in an expiratory articulation as three syllables. Again, silence. Once more the resident tried, in vain, before leaving the room, to return with an Asian woman who repeated the words in the patient's native tongue. The Asian man was not confused. He simply did not speak English - a fact that had eluded his doctors before seeking psychiatric consultation.

Perry was psychologically and emotionally mature and felt no need of psychiatry and/or psychiatrists. He was not oblivious, as was Dr. Soup, to the consensus of opinion that the main point of psychiatry in a setting of depressive news is to dissuade patients of suicidal notions that might attend conceptualization of death with dignity. He felt entitled to any sense of depression provoked by the brutal pronouncement of impending death and responded simply that he did not need psychiatric evaluation. He told me and our sons of his refusal and we registered our objection with the staff. He was not confused or overwhelmed by feelings of being burdensome to his family, did not wish for an accelerated end to ease their burden, wanted more time that newer treatments for his cancer might afford, and lacked not for antidepressants.

But Dr. Soup returned the next morning and badgered Perry that an encounter with a psychiatrist would do him good, cryptically writing that the patient agreed to see a psychiatrist which, in fact the record memorialized elsewhere that he had refused. When I confronted him with the fact that both the patient and his family had stated they did not wish for an encounter with a psychiatrist, Dr. Soup arrogantly maintained that it was his right, not that of either patient or family, to determine and proceed as he dictated. Pressed, he admitted that he had not read Perry's chart and was unfamiliar with the history or, in fact, the patient, but this was unimportant because he had a feel for these things.

The consultative note provides clear evidence that Perry one-upped the psychiatrist and took charge of the interview. He began by stating he did not want family members present, followed by a description of a wonderful full life lived with meaning, then expressed his pride and enjoyment in his exceptional family, after which he denied having a low mood, thoughts of self-harm or death wishes, and finally he indicated contented anticipation of his life in the world to come. The psychiatrist's notes state that the patient had "organized thought processes with good insight and intact judgment."

Chapter 28

AND SO IT GOES

When he returned to Dr. Slobber at the outpatient clinic, still awaiting MDV-3100, the PSA was 750. He had been throwing up, had no appetite, was not sleeping, and had increased leg and butt pain. He asked for results of circulating tumor cell analysis performed during the IMC-temsirolimus protocol, and wondered if the pain came from nerve inflammation. Dr. Slobber ignored his questions. Her note states significant impairment in ambulation, hemoglobin and platelets are further decreased, an emergency MRI shows extensive blastic osseous metastases involving lower spine, pelvis and proximal femurs, persistent cortical destruction, extraosseous extension from bilateral metastases in the pubic bones, no acute fracture, a caudal compromise without cord impingement at T7, and disease impinging the L5, S1, S2 and S3 nerve roots.

She sent him to Urgent Care to exclude disease that needs radiation and for neurology evaluation and wrote that if workup was negative he should return for initiation of docetaxel, dispensing with his query about MDV-3100 with a terse: "It's not available" adding in her notes, "the patient's physician wife not present but was alerted to the issues." The alert came some hours later from the Urgent Care physician who informed me that my husband would be admitted to the hospital on the neurology service. He was discharged after two days with gabapentin and tramadol for nerve pain and for sleep, and an appointment in the neurology clinic ten days later.

He didn't make that neurology appointment because before the scheduled date he returned to Dr. Slobber for his first dose of docetaxel, soon after which he had to go back to Urgent Care with terrible diarrhea and a huge hematoma on his left shin from a fall, which never healed. Again Dr. Slobber wrote: "Wife notified." Again the notification came from an Urgent Care physician telling me my husband was there. He received two units of red blood cells for an abysmal hemoglobin of 7.7, platelet count also noted as dismally low, and was sent home to return for follow-up at the outpatient clinic, which would be for his next dose of docetaxel.

In the interim, we took our annual summer vacation in the Poconos with sons and grandchildren, but Perry was miserable the whole time, barely able to ambulate and with continuous pain. He revived a couple of times, one memorably during a transcontinental phone conversation with his life-long friend who had been residing in Israel for a couple of decades. Perry did his best to engage in their usual geopolitical interchanges but avoided questions regarding his disease and physical state.

Chapter 29

NOT A DREAM

"Move over!" Perry exclaimed a few nights after we returned home, pushing forcefully against my body. "You're taking up too much room, I'm going to fall out of the boat!"

I pushed back saying that there was no boat, we were in bed, to no avail.
"My mother and father are too big," he went on, "there's not enough room for them, they have to get out of the boat."

I tried to wake him, telling him he was dreaming. But when he pushed a couple more times and continued rambling about a maritime disaster I realized he was hallucinating. That morning he had been to another oncologist to receive his second dose of docetaxel while Dr. Slobber was away on a cruise, and had pleaded for something that would help him sleep. The oncologist obliged, prescribing Ambien. One of the most popular drugs for insomnia, Ambien is notorious for its side effects, including frequent reports of hallucinations. This likely pertains to part of its chemical structure, deliberately modeled on LSD because of its ability to penetrate and be active in the brain. Other risky side effects include sleep driving and having sex, neither of which Perry attempted. I managed to arouse him from sleep and keep him wakeful for a spell, and the rest of the night passed without incident. I noted to myself that he shouldn't take Ambien again.

Chapter 30

RADIATION

The next evening he was back at Urgent Care. The pain was worse. He was assessed by multiple physicians of various ilk, including some from radiation oncology who rendered the opinion that he was a "good candidate for palliative radiation." Their note reads: "discussed risks, benefits, alternatives, rationales for radiation therapy with patient and his wife, answered many questions to their satisfaction..." *blah, blah, blah* – This was shocking to read since I, the wife, had left Urgent Care to get Perry the milk shake he requested from an ice cream parlor a couple of blocks away.

I returned about 30 minutes later to learn from my husband that the radiation oncology service had been to see him. They said the side effects were minimal and they could protect him against them. They then put an informed consent in front of him to sign, which he did after they insisted that his wife wasn't necessary.

The radiation treatment had onerous side effects, the most distressing being horrendous diarrhea. Perry withstood without complaint this and every other physical and emotional invasion, waiting and hoping for positive response to the radiation. Nor did he complain when abruptly moved to another room because the one he was in was scheduled for redecoration. Visited by some hospital functionary who asked how he liked the new room, which had been recently redecorated, Perry perfunctorily answered that it was lovely. This resulted in persistent irksome phone calls and letters to his wife soliciting donations. I found this an ill-timed effrontery in light of Perry's physical incapacitance and the noncaring medical staff. Sick as he was, he retained his sense of humor, and was totally receptive to my climbing into his hospital bed each evening. He would put his arm around me as we watched the nightly news and other programs on TV.

He was visited regularly by a physical therapist with the goal of transferring him to an acute rehab center at a nearby hospital. This was accomplished close to three weeks after his first inpatient radiation treatment. Transfer to rehab had been arranged for the very afternoon of the day of his last radiation treatment.

Chapter 31

TO REHAB AND BACK

Weak but responding to the rehab program, he developed a fever of unknown origin. This prompted blood draws which revealed very low hemoglobin and platelets, not at all surprising given the course of radiation and the fact that his blood counts were already quite low the very day he was transferred. Rehab knew not what to do, and sent him back to the famous cancer hospital where, in yet another series of scans, an incidental small subdural hematoma was found, undoubtedly related to the low platelets. As to the dismal blood counts Dr. Slobber commented: "No one expected this."

What did she expect after massive doses of radiation and the alarming blood counts on the day he was sent to rehab?

He soon developed other problems. His undernourished state was reflected in low serum albumin which, coupled with a low serum sodium, gave rise to fluid accumulation in his lungs and extremities. It was early July, traditionally considered to be a bad time in any hospital because that is the month of the influx of raw interns fresh out of medical school with paltry clinical acumen or experience. Perry questioned the one who was assigned to his case who argued strenuously that his condition required drainage of fluid from the pleural cavity - a pulmonologist would be consulted - telling me the same when I came to visit later that day. I asked to speak with Dr. Slobber. Instead I got a badgering call from the intern saying that it was beneath the attending's position to call. He was "The Doctor" and his opinion reigned. He noted in the record: "The wife made inappropriate requests."

The staff pulmonologist did not assign communication with family to an underling and had the courtesy to telephone me after seeing my husband in consultation. His opinion, coinciding with mine, was that draining fluid from the chest by thoracentesis would be of brief and limited benefit. Since the pleural fluid primarily resulted from inadequate osmotic pressure due to the very low serum albumin, pushing fluid out of the vascular system into extracellular spaces, it would soon re-accumulate. He recommended vigorous diuresis to eliminate excess fluid and only after such, or unless infection was suspected – which was not – would thoracentesis be indicated. And indeed, that approach worked.

Chapter 32

OTHER UNDERLINGS

The rotating attending physicians, although more experienced than the recently graduated interns, were dependent functionaries. They were cognizant of their relative status in the well-established staff hierarchy and fearful of reprimand by the more senior attendings. I privately referred to them with pseudonyms epitomizing their personas.

Dr. Ratchett was dubbed with this moniker because of her martinet behavior and unfailing attention to hospital protocol minutiae that evoked the so named nurse in *One Flew over the Cuckoo's Nest*. Incapable of the least modicum of humanity, on one occasion she abruptly ordered an MRI without forewarning. Perry was inexplicably wheeled off for his second MRI of the day, but returned to his room forthwith when an astute technician realized that twenty-four hours were needed to clear the previous imaging tracer.

He had so many MRIs that I was persuaded that the team viewed them as a profit center. Salaries of hospital-employed physicians are related to the income they generate, which makes one wonder. Logic dictates that the paltry $25 or so Medicare payment allowance for a physician hospital or office visit, at a charge of several fold more, cannot support an oncologist's six-figure salary. One cannot help pondering if some reward transpires in the accounting of physician service for productivity in this regard. Or was it fear of malpractice litigation that inspired ordering unnecessary procedures to provide proof that everything possible was done.

The moniker Dr. Romania suited the man because he was born and raised in Romania. In his late thirties, it was clear that he learned well the lessons of a repressive dictatorial regime. He was incapable of contesting the authoritative voice of his hierarchical superiors.

The horribly flawed conduct of the medical staff was characterized by a dispassionate modus operandi of infantilization and dehumanization of my husband, myself and in those final months, our sons. Every question was met with disdain or denial, overridden with smug dismissal, and countered with glib self-justification.

My husband's chart is replete with notes of interactions in which various findings and procedures were purportedly presented to the patient and his family, yet no physician on the prostate oncology service ever offered anything other than platitudes or obfuscating medical jargon, deliberately circumventing meaningful discussion or response to specific questions. The eldest viewed Dr. Slobber, the physician of record in charge, as negligent and drew interesting parallels with the Cambodian genocidal maniac, Pol Pot who, when interviewed some eighteen years after presiding over Cambodia's killing fields, declared 'My conscience is clear,' and with Hannah Arendt's description of Adolf Eichmann going to the gallows 'with great dignity.'

Chapter 33

THE REIGNING QUEEN

A week after Perry's transfer back to the famous cancer hospital, our eldest son encountered Dr. Slobber. She was serving her two weeks turn as inpatient attending. He related to me his total frustration at her jargon and avoidance of addressing his legitimate concerns and questions. But her note of this encounter, with a shrewd eye to potential consequence if reviewed by a third party, distorts what actually transpired:

"I just spent 36.26 minutes on the floor with patient's son, in the presence of the nursing supervisor and the nursing manager, who he had contacted regarding his dissatisfaction with hospital care and lack of nutritional input. I chronicled the hospital course and the rationale for all consultations by various services, but the son cut me short and wanted to focus on specific issues including rehab, well-being and future treatment. I explained that the patient had a subdural hematoma requiring one week of platelet transfusion, the plan would then be to observe and if in the 50-60K range consider a return to rehab for improvement on deconditioning issues. I told him that the patient had been using inhalation spirometry in addition to getting chest PT, nutrition has been seeing patient regularly, we have been encouraging the patient to do more for himself, and that his father is definitely eating, but that the cancer itself could cause decreased oral intake secondary to soluble factors which suppresses the appetite. Overall the patient remains stable. No treatment is planned as long as patient is thrombocytopenic and despite available chemotherapeutic agents I am disinclined to risk further marrow suppression. I also informed him that we are addressing psychological well-being, but I can't force patient to it if he declines."

If he were eating why were his trays returned untouched? Why were the high protein shakes accumulating in the refrigerator?

His only nutrition was what we brought in, hoping to entice him with something rich in protein that he liked, such as sashimi - or the few high protein shakes we personally coached him to drink. Notwithstanding Dr. Slobber's remarkable need to stipulate, to the second, the time spent in discussion with our son, more mind-boggling was her deliberate omission of the fact that she had sent Perry to Rehab with low platelets, had watched his disease progress, and had withheld requested treatment. Michael's account to me after this encounter was one of incredulity at her avoidance of every issue raised with a tirade of medical terms that he did not understand and which she refused to answer by interruption and reversion to her lecture stance. Frustrated, he told her that he did not find the conversation satisfactory and that she needed to speak with me.

After days of requests to discuss the status and treatment plan I got a telephone message that Dr. Slobber would be able to meet with me at 6:30pm. It was a carefully arranged meeting. She appeared in my husband's room a few minutes late with a pronounced tell of discomfort, accompanied by the head of nursing who stood mute, but was not the only witness to the conversation. Perry was there. I was there. And so was Michael. Perry had developed a cold a few days earlier and had been placed in an isolation room, requiring mask and gown, although all cultures of every body fluid had proved negative.

Dr. Slobber embarked on an offensive and demeaning discourse, referring to Perry as if nonexistent and incapable of making decisions for himself. She called his upper respiratory tract infection a "drippy schnozzola," and brooked no questions, allowed no discussion. She rudely and insistently raised her voice to cut off any and all attempts at medical or other reasonable interchange. She exuded chastisement and threat that Michael and I were daring to question her and pronounced that challenging her authority was beyond our purviews and would be to my husband's detriment. Michael calmly stated that we wished only to engage in meaningful dialogue with her in the hope of accruing to his father's benefit. At this point Dr. Slobber hunched her shoulders and aggressively moved sideways, thrust her face into Michael's and said with a deliberate threatening air: "I will call security to have you removed from the room."

Michael calmly responded that he merely wanted our questions answered, which her obfuscating jargon failed to do. Dr. Slobber inched even closer to Michael, reinforcing a physical threat and repeating her verbal one. Noting my husband's obvious distress at Dr. Slobber's behavior, and hoping to defuse her hostility and arrogant behavior, I asked Michael to let it go. I still hoped that we could have a civilized discussion that would accomplish some of the purpose of the meeting. But alas, Dr. Slobber persisted in her harassment of Michael, continued her abusive proclamations, cut off further discussion, and swept from the room.

"Wow, she really gave it to you," Perry said when Dr. Slobber left the room. But what the unassailable and credentialed Dr. Slobber entered in his chart was quite different from what actually transpired.

It said that she had met with the patient's son who criticized her for having discussed psychiatry with his father. It then said that when she tried to pursue it, the son approached her in an aggressive manner, that she asked him not to tell her what to say and that his mother kept saying to him 'let it go.' She noted that son has been looking toward social worker for emotional support of his father but we learned from the patient that he did not appreciate social worker visits and wanted it to stop. All questions were answered to satisfaction of wife and son. Disposition was discussed and plan is to see what platelet count will do after Friday. Strategies about treatment were discussed, as was a need for a hematologic safety margin.

The entry is the epitome of an institutional employee who is well-attuned to potential legal ramifications of anything in the patient's chart. Her note is a carefully honed distortion by a smooth-talker confident in her unaccountability, misrepresenting every aspect of her own behavior, as well as of that of everyone else present. She knew how to parse a self-protective account and cast aspersions on the patient's family in a hailstorm of fabrications and accusatory diatribes. She twisted my husband's articulated wishes that he had neither need nor desire for social worker or psychiatrist, turning them topsy-turvy to insinuate fault on his part.

Chapter 34

NO RECOURSE

Perry knew that the Phase III trial of MDV3100 was stopped early upon showing clinically meaningful and statistically significant improvement in overall survival. It was now available under the name Xtandia. He also knew that the drug was developed at the famous cancer hospital. Its Chief of Genitourinary Oncology was a principal investigator and its leading proponent. He well-remembered Dr. Slobber's pronouncement a couple of months earlier that it "was the drug for him", and he had agreed.

I witnessed several times when, speaking of MDV3100, my husband told Dr. Romania "I want it." Dr. Romania always gave the same response: "We could talk about it." He really didn't want to talk about it; he was low man on the totem pole and he could only do or say what Dr. Slobber allowed him to do or say.

Exasperated we wrote a letter and delivered it by hand to the Chief of the Genitourinary Oncology Service and the Senior Vice President and Hospital Administrator. We copied it to Dr. Slobber and the other oncologists who had been in-patient attendings and asked that a copy be inserted into his chart - *which it was not.*

The letter laid out Perry's ardent desire to receive this latest drug which had been approved by the FDA for treatment of metastatic castration resistant prostate cancer in patients previously treated with docetaxel. Perry fit the criteria and he wanted it badly.

A small incidence (less than 1%) of patients in the trial had experienced seizure, and it was clear to us that the reason for refusal by famous cancer hospital was fear that any such incident would detract from market acceptance of their drug. The letter addressed this remote eventuality and articulated his right to receive this drug.

We write to make this urgent request that Perry be offered a prescription for MDV3100.

He fully understands, as do we, that one side effect of MDV3100, reported in roughly 1% of patients in a recent experimental trial, is seizure. He also understands, as do we, that his attending physicians at the hospital believe that his risk is higher, and for that reason have expressed reluctance to prescribe this treatment. Nonetheless, under the accepted canons of medical ethics, the patient has a fundamental right of self-decision. The decision whether or not to pursue MDV3100, after full disclosure of relevant risks, belongs to the patient. We ask that you work with the patient and his family so that he may provide written, informed consent that places with him and him alone, full responsibility for the risk of an adverse event.

Perry has metastatic prostate cancer and has received two cycles of docetaxel-based chemotherapy. Recent studies have shown that MDV3100 extends the median overall survival of men with metastatic prostate cancer who have already been treated with at least one cycle of docetaxel-based chemotherapy by an average of 5 months. The patient thus falls precisely within the class of persons for whom this drug was developed and for whom it is recommended under accelerated FDA approval.

We, and Perry, understand that there is a reported 1% incidence of seizures as a side-effect. We, and the named patient, also understand that the attending doctors believe that he may be at higher risk for this side effect because of evidence of prior small but stable subdural hematoma. This is an important starting point for medical decision-making, but it is not the end. We, and the named patient, believe there is a reasonable ground for disagreement as to whether this finding places him at a risk higher than 1%, for reasons mentioned. Regardless, even assuming the risk is higher than 1%, that does not mean the risk is not worth taking. A seizure is a serious side-effect but is not inherently fatal. Balanced against that risk, moreover, is the substantial probability that if no action is taken, both Perry's life expectancy, and his quality of life expectancy, may be quite short.

We also know, and Perry's attending physicians have acknowledged, that it is part of their medical practice – and indeed part of sound medical practice – to prescribe courses of treatment with significant risk.

We are at cross-roads. The choice is whether to sit idly by and let a horrible disease take its course unabated, or whether to pursue a treatment course that provides the only known hope of a better outcome, within a degree of risk that Perry is willing to tolerate. We, and Perry, do not believe that he should be forced to take the first path by default, when another course of action exists. We do not have the luxury of time to study this issue further. With every day that passes Perry's cancer advances."

Separately, Perry provided a signed, dated and witnessed informed consent to receive the drug. He stated that he had been fully counseled by the hospital medical staff concerning a course of treatment involving MDV3100. They had discussed with him his diagnosis; the nature and purpose of the proposed treatment; the risks and benefits of this proposed treatment; alternatives (regardless of their cost or the extent to which the treatment options are covered by health insurance); the risks and benefits of the alternative treatment or procedure; and the risks and benefits of not receiving or undergoing a treatment or procedure. He had been provided a full opportunity to ask questions and have answered any questions he asked. He further stated that he understood that in an experimental trial, 1% of patients reported seizure as a side effect of the drug and that, because of a history of subdural hematoma, he may be at a significantly higher risk for seizure if he took MDV3100 and that, having weighed the alternatives and having received full and complete disclosure from hospital medical staff of the attendant risks, he wished to pursue this course of treatment.

He accepted full, sole and complete responsibility for this decision.

The response to the letter and informed consent was a visit by the medical ethicist who had been commissioned to review his request. She moved to his bed and whispered closely into his ear, asking if he wanted the drug. He responded clearly: "Yes, yes, yes."

Soon thereafter, Michael and I were summoned to a meeting with Dr. Slobber and more than half a dozen others, all sitting with forced pleasantness across from us and at each end of the conference table. I recognized one nurse and the patient advocate who had the gall to tell Michael: "We are watching you for your misbehavior" - as witnessed by our Rabbi, who voiced outrage at violation of the most fundamental rules of compassionate care.

Dr. Slobber expounded on risks, stating: "We don't know what neurologic or other side effects there might be, we will not give this drug." No one else said a word.

What is the ethics committee? Who were these people who refused to identify themselves?
By what right can they hold a closed enclave, a self-appointed arbitrary Star Chamber to determine a patient's fate? To whom are they accountable? Where is the right of appeal to judgment?

Chapter 35

WHAT OTHERS SAY

In his book *The Death of Cancer,* Vincent DeVita, former head of the National Cancer Institute and subsequently physician-in-chief at Memorial Sloan Kettering, described his dogged pursuit to keep a good friend alive after relapse following radical prostatectomy. At one point he tried to get the man enrolled in an experimental drug protocol that dictated a fixed number of doses, advocating a longer course which required permission from the hospital's institutional review board, and was denied. In subsequent unremitting pursuit, he succeeded in enrolling his friend in several other trials with other drugs, but failed in his endeavor for abiraterone, subsequently shown to significantly prolong life and win approval from the FDA, because of some inflexibility in enrollment criteria.

Chapter 36

DONE WITH HIM

Within a day after the meeting with the ethics committee Dr. Slobber transferred Perry to another hospital for blood transfusion. She provided the name of an oncologist on the staff of that hospital who promptly came to see him. He said he would be Perry's physician and would prescribe MDV-3100 (Xtandia), telling him they were "giant pills," asking him if he thought he could swallow them, and if he was sure he wanted them. Perry again answered: "Yes, yes."

Alas, it was too late. Transferred to a subacute rehab facility, Perry's course had a rapidly progressive downward spiral that was alleviated with morphine. On the night of Hurricane Sandy I called our sons into the room when his respirations changed. We sat together watching his final breaths.

The one physician who exhibited grace and compassion in those final days was the oncologist who prescribed Xtandia. There was not a peep from anyone at famous cancer hospital.

Chapter 37

REFLECTIONS

I am no stranger to the physician's need to avoid emotional involvement, to shield oneself from the pain of loss when incurable disease has run its course, to cover looming grief with cold clinical competency. But I believe my patients and their families felt I was humane and caring - if not, why would they invite me to their homes to sit Shiva, or occasionally send heartfelt notes and even gifts after the death of their loved one?

Not so for the team at the famous cancer hospital. Even a customary morning greeting was rarely delivered. Marching into the room for patient rounds, the attending physician stood mute, maintaining a steely face of non-involvement while one of the phalanx of underlings delivered the day's pronouncements in clipped, chipper tones.

Around his 90th birthday Dr. Arnold Relman, long-term editor of the New England Journal of Medicine and emeritus Professor of Medicine at Harvard, suffered a fall. His injury was compounded by various complications, and his status was precarious. After eleven touch-and-go days of acute care, he was sufficiently stable for transfer to a less acute facility. About eight months after the initial injury, rehabilitated and carefully assuming daily activities, he lucidly recounted his experience in an essay in the New York Times. He lauded the expert emergency medical treatment and the excellence of the nursing attention, making special notice of the importance of the latter. But he also made sharp observations on medicine as practiced in a hospital setting and on the teams of physicians who visited on daily rounds. He noted that they spent most of their time hovering outside his room, studying and discussing the computer data of laboratory and imaging findings. Their interactions with the patient were short and perfunctory.

The accuracy of those comments totally resonated with me. Very clear memory of my husband's ordeal, coupled with combing through his voluminous hospital records and his personal files, left me with little doubt about Dr. Relman's sharp observations. Physicians' notes are primarily written by the lowliest house officers and largely consist of regurgitated laboratory data and radiographic reports. There is little mention of the patient per se. Attending staff are loath to make entries in a patient's chart and appear to do so only when someone has called something into question, and are careless in putting their signature on reports dictated by underlings.

Chapter 38

AFTER

The things my husband left behind are illogically meaningful. I see him in the drawers full of underwear and socks, racks of ties, shirts and suits hanging in his closet, shelves of tennis outfits and gear, innumerable jackets, and a veritable store of baseball caps in the front closet.

In the winter after his initial surgery my husband made an uncharacteristically expensive purchase at Barney's of a cashmere coat which he had seen an acquaintance wearing and had much admired. The elegant dark coat, perfectly fitted to his tall stature and erect carriage now hung in a closet, above the two pairs of costly shoes languishing in their boxes - size twelve and a half, triple A - never worn. They had been too snug when he tried them on at home and I accompanied him to the store for stretching. These objects left behind echoed my husband's resolve to survive in the face of his diagnosis. I attempted to rid myself of the pain they evoked by giving them to my daughter-in-law to sell on e-bay.

For a long time his closet and dresser drawers remained full, save for a few things our sons accepted such as some shirts, a couple of ties they took in a pinch after sleeping over and being without one for work the next day, and a red and blue striped sailor jacket with a dashing crest purchased in Sorrento the year before he died. The gold bracelet I gave my husband in the seventies when such things were in fashion I gifted to our eldest son, the elementary school awarded gold-plated chain with his name strung in elongated fashion I gave to our eldest grandson as a personal remembrance of his Papa Perry.

My personal grief after loss of my husband is private and unique to the person that he was and that I am. The demonstration, too late for my husband, that the very drugs he was denied prolong survival, is good news for others. Not fair, he was a good man..

The memories of his dignified life and the undignified care perpetrated at the famous cancer hospital remain.

Chapter 39

FROM ON HIGH

The U.S. Preventative Services Task Force recommended in 2012 that men stop getting routine PSA tests for detection of prostate cancer. The report cited data from large scale studies in the U.S. and Europe as evidence that the benefit of PSA and early treatment ranges from 0 to 1 deaths avoided per 1000 men screened. This was accompanied by a lengthy discussion of the potential harms resulting from an elevated PSA value, including excessive worry, overdiagnosis and hence overtreatment, the usual therapeutic approaches of surgery, radiation or androgen deprivation bringing risks of long-term adverse effects such as erectile, urinary and bowel dysfunction.

The recommendation provoked much discussion, refutation, and differences of opinion. The American Society of Clinical Oncologists concluded that PSA screening could reduce deaths from prostate cancer by 20 percent in men with a life expectancy of more than 10 years. Rather than blanket abandonment of PSA testing, they supported commencement of PSA screening at about age 50, and encouraged patient education of the pluses and minuses of the PSA test as well as consideration of factors such as family history and patient age.

One sage commentator noted that no member of the task force was engaged in clinical care of patients with prostate cancer. Comprised of primary care pediatricians, family physicians, internists, nurses, obstetricians/gynecologists, epidemiologists and statisticians, the interests of the individual members are described as decision modeling and evaluation, clinical epidemiology, the prevention of high-risk behaviors in adolescents, and the prevention of disability in the elderly.

The notion of ill-advisedness of PSA testing in men with life expectancy less than 10 years stems from the likelihood of death from cardiac, pulmonary or other morbid disease - rather than from prostate cancer in that time frame. Survival studies often employ retrospective analysis of information gleaned from death certificates, which may not accurately reflect the cause of death.

Apparently appreciating this problem, the house doctor who signed Perry's death certificate consulted with me when he found that prostate cancer was not accepted as cause of death. The only primary cause that the system would accept was cardiac arrest and, with that entry, the only secondary cause that the system would accept was heart disease. He stated that the system wouldn't allow entry of prostate cancer.

Of course, everyone dies of cardiac arrest, but not everyone's heart stops because of intrinsic heart disease. Perry had neither history nor evidence of heart disease, and had enviable blood pressures, cholesterol levels and the like his entire life. He enjoyed excellent cardiac function and physical stamina until his terminal days.

To ascribe cause of death to cardiac disease was false reporting, and I vigorously objected. Unable to persuade me, the physician left the room for some time to research the system, listened to my suggestions, and made the more appropriate entries of anemia and prostate cancer in the death certificate. At about five grams, his hemoglobin was insufficient to sustain life and was due to bone marrow invasion by prostate cancer - which could be respectively coded as secondary and tertiary cause of death.

As I sat waiting for the house physician's return, I contemplated the dubious accuracy of the many reports concluding that upwards of 80 percent of men with prostate cancer died of something else. The telling feature of the argument in the anti-PSA screening camp is that "statistics" indicate that most patients with this malignancy die of "other disease," notably listed as "cardiac." Hence the notion that intervention for an elevated PSA does not "save lives." The 2017 recommendations for upper limits of normal blood pressure are reminiscent of this argument in that yes, cardiovascular events may be lessened by adhering to the new standard, but at the risk of raising the likelihood of potentially lethal falls from drug-induced hypotension, prompting the astute commentary that death after such would be attributed to "complications of an accidental fall" and misleading statistics indicating that cardiovascular death was prevented.

This is exactly why I deemed it important that what caused my husband's death be accurate. He died from prostate cancer.

Definitions

CAT Scan - X-ray image made using computerized axial tomography

Cauda Equina Syndrome – compression of nerve roots at the end of the spinal canal

Diamox – drug affects acid-base balance

Fentanyl – an opioid

Gleason Score – estimate of potential aggressivity of prostate cancer based on cellular characteristics

Hemoglobin – red blood cell protein that carries oxygen

Hyperplasia – enlargement of an organ

Iatrogenic – caused by medical examination or treatment

Inguinal - groin

LHRH – Luteinizing Releasing Hormone

Lymphocele – a collection of lymphatic fluid

Lyse - break

MRI – Imaging that uses a magnetic field and radio waves

PET scan – positron emission tomography imaging

Prostascint – Imaging that uses a radioactive molecule coupled to an antibody that attaches to prostate-specific membrane antigen

Pulmonary embolus – blood clot in lung

PSA – Prostate-Specific Antigen

Retroperitoneal – behind the peritoneum, the membrane covering abdominal organs

www.ingramcontent.com/pod-product-compliance
Lightning Source LLC
Chambersburg PA
CBHW030444220526
45464CB00006B/2414